D1430041

Working My Way Back to Me

A PRIMER FOR STROKE SURVIVORS,
FAMILY MEMBERS, AND CAREGIVERS

Lincoln Krochmal, MD

FINN-PHYLLIS
PRESS

Contents

Foreword...5

Introduction 9

01: The Recovery Road Begins 13

02: Regaining Freedom and Independence 27

03: Depression 31

04: The Birth of Dr. K.......................................37

05: Find Humor in the Mundane......................43

06: The Therapist Ticket...................................49

07: Preparing to Go Home 53

08: Rehab Fatigue 57

09: Keeping a Positive Attitude.........................61

10: Home At Last..69

11: Regaining Freedom at the DMV.................75

12: Re-Immersion...79

13: Bye Bye Wheelchair 85

14: East Meets West 87

15: Where I Stand Today..................................93

Top 12 Directives for Patients..........................97

Appendix 98

Glossary..101

Acknowledgements...107

About the Author 109

To my amazing family—my wife, Lana; my son, Noah; and my daughter, Natalie. Without your love, support, and care, I would not be alive today.

"Physician, Heal Thyself."
—Jesus, *The Gospel of St. Luke*

Every book should have a reason and purpose for being written, whether to entertain or to document, propose, inform, or educate. This book is written for the latter reason, and to tell my story as a physician committed to healing himself from a stroke. The intended audience includes survivors of strokes and non-fatal traumatic brain injuries (TBIs) and their families, loved ones, caregivers, and therapists. Many books already exist in this space (and are referenced in the appendix), all of which I have read and learned from.

However, as a stroke survivor who is also a physician, I believe I have a unique perspective that is worth sharing, as it emphasizes truth and reality over hearsay and misperceptions regarding the immediate period after injury, the near- and longer-term recovery period, and the long-term outlook for stroke and TBI patients.

One question I'm frequently asked is regarding why I

survived this severe stroke, as the odds were certainly against me. In fact, the doctors said the bleed was so extensive that it should have killed me. Therefore, I've pondered why I survived, and it's a difficult question to answer. Was it by some divine intervention that I was spared so that I could do something to help others such as write this book to help new stroke survivors and their families? Or lead a stroke survivor group? Or see my daughter get married, have a recommitment ceremony with my wife, and then enjoy my one and only grandchild? Or was it so that I could prove that I could (and would) walk, drive, and work again? To show my wife and children that I was strong, the head of the household, and would not let a stroke destroy the father and husband they had known? Counsel new stroke survivors that they could get better as I did, provided they were willing to work hard on their recovery? I am of course not completely sure why I survived, but I did, and I've been determined ever since to prove many of the naysayers wrong with respect to one's ability to live a truly meaningful life after a stroke.

My goal is for this book to be an invaluable primer for an audience longing to know what has happened to the patient, how he or she is likely to be feeling, and how this event will impact their collective lives. Of course, each patient's experience will be different. The timelines that I experienced may or may not correlate with yours or those of your loved one, but I'm including them to give you an idea of one person's experience, since I know one of your burning questions will likely be "How long until...?"

Most importantly, I aim to provide guidance on preparing for the challenging road ahead. I trust that this book will be as helpful and informative to others as it would have been for me in achieving my goal of reclaiming my life and healing myself after this unexpected and life-changing event.

INTRODUCTION

I awoke on a Sunday morning (September 5th, 2010) to a typical Northern California day, ready to wash up in the bathroom following a Viagra-enhanced night of wonderful love making with my wife, Lana.

Lana and I met during the summer of 1969, following my second year of medical school. I was enrolled at the Marquette School of Medicine in Milwaukee (now known as the Medical College of Wisconsin). During the summer between the second and third year of medical school, medical students were permitted to work as externs in a hospital under the supervision of a physician, and as luck would have it, I was able to secure a position at Mount Sinai (a private hospital in Milwaukee), where Lana was the head Emergency Room nurse. An externship included time rotating through various services in the hospital, including the ER, surgery, general medicine, pediatrics, and orthopedics. Little did I realize at the time how significant the summer of '69 would be in my life.

My first assignment was to be in the emergency room. After showing up on the first day, I noticed a beautiful brunette nurse who immediately captivated my attention and my heart. I introduced myself to her and learned that her name was Lana. She was the head nurse and would supervise me during my two-week-long rotation in the ER, along with the ER physician. Being with Lana daily was an amazing experience. I truly believed I had met my future wife, so our courtship began in earnest. For me, it was truly love at first sight! Although I was supposed to rotate to other areas of the hospital after those two weeks in the ER, I managed to find ways to remain close to her department for the entire summer.

I soon came to realize what an excellent nurse Lana was, as she taught me many procedures, such as how to start an IV, examine acutely traumatized patients, and generally function in an ER, never knowing what was coming through the door. This experience served me quite well when I later spent two years as a general physician working on an Indian reservation in Montana.

As Lana and I began dating, we had memorable picnic outings after work along the shores of Lake Michigan in the beautiful parks that lined Lake Shore Drive. Love blossomed and we married in 1971, just prior to my graduation from medical school. We delayed our honeymoon until the summer following graduation and then spent three weeks in Mexico before heading to Boston, where I would intern in the US Public Health Hospital. This marked the beginning of our life's sojourn. I am happy to report we have been married for over fifty years and are still very much enjoying our life's partnership, even with all its unexpected twists and turns.

While standing at the sink, I began to feel unsteady, like a ship in rough waters. I had no headache or pain, but I felt as though I might fall, so I grabbed the front edge of the sink where the overflow holes are located, and very gently lowered myself to the bathroom floor. I called for my wife, who was able to see me from our bed, who immediately came to my side on the floor. As a well-trained emergency room nurse, she could see that I was unable to move my left arm or leg, my speech was somewhat slurred, and my face had drooped a bit on the left side. She quickly and correctly diagnosed that I was having a stroke.

I, on the other hand, was not quite sure what was happening. But the longer I lay on the floor, the more her diagnosis of a stroke seemed to be correct. Given that I had no pain anywhere, I knew I was not having a heart attack!

I begged her to help me get back into bed. Thankfully, she instead covered me with a blanket, made me comfortable, and went to call 911 to get help. I could hear her arguing with the operator after requesting that an ambulance be dispatched to the house. The operator was questioning how Lana knew what was going on with me; apparently, they get a lot of calls that aren't true emergencies. My wife explained that she was an emergency room nurse who had seen stroke patients and was sure from my symptoms that a stroke was what I was experiencing. She demanded that they quit arguing with her and send an ambulance. They did.

I'm so grateful for her knowledge and her quick response. Had I gone back to bed as I wanted to do (while she knew not to let me do), I would have died.

Soon, the fire department and an ambulance with EMTs arrived. Once the paramedics were in our bathroom with us, they continued to ask me (over and over again) the same questions in order to assess my mental status and orientation: "What day of the week is it?" "What is the date?" "Who is the president?" "What is your name and address?"

After several rounds of these questions, I began giving them the answers before they were even asked, which everyone thought was funny. They brought in a gurney, transferred me onto a sheet and then onto the gurney, and took me down our front stairs to the ambulance. This would be my first experience riding in an ambulance—as a patient, anyway.

CHAPTER ONE

The Recovery Road Begins

STROKE FACT

Every stroke or TBI is unique in its recovery period.

I graduated medical school in 1971 and subsequently worked for a year in Boston in an internship. I then spent two years working in general practice on an Indian reservation in Montana as a volunteer in the U.S. Public Health Service, then trained for three years at the University of Missouri in Columbia to become a dermatologist. Following completion of my residency, I opened my practice in Billings, Montana, where I saw 150,000 patients over the following eight years.

In 1983, I decided to join a pharmaceutical company, Bristol-Myers, in order to conduct research and development for new therapies for skin diseases. At that time, I stopped seeing patients on a regular basis so I could devote one hundred percent of my time to research.

During a ski trip in Montana in 1981, I dislocated my left shoulder, which subsequently required surgical repair some years later. That was the first time I underwent the process of being treated as a patient (other than a short hospital stay for kidney stones). Since my time as a patient was quite limited while having my shoulder repaired, it was not until suffering the stroke that I really began to understand life from the perspective of a patient rather than a physician. The transition was challenging; it was difficult for me to suddenly be placed in the position of taking orders and direction from physicians instead of directing my patients on how to treat their skin conditions.

The ambulance ride to the closest hospital was thankfully quite short, yet I vividly remember feeling every bump, pothole, and speed bump along the way, all of which were most uncomfortable. They would not permit any family to accompany me in the ambulance, so Lana drove herself separately after calling our daughter, Natalie, (who lived nearby) to inform her of what had happened.

While in the ambulance, I listened to everything that was being said in an effort to understand what was happening to me, but the noise of the siren was overwhelming. The ride seemed endless and was tortuous, not knowing what was going on. I naturally feared the worst since, as a physician, I knew that a percentage of strokes patients die shortly after having a stroke. Not being able to move my left arm and leg combined with an inability to speak clearly left me feeling a bit panicky.

The EMTs continued to check me cognitively in terms of

being oriented to time, place, and person. I didn't engage in any idle chatter with them as they continued to monitor my vital signs. I tried to relax, but it was very difficult to do so. I kept hoping the ambulance wouldn't get into an accident as it sped through intersections on the way to the hospital.

As Natalie and Lana drove to the hospital, Lana was in total shock and filled with emotions about my condition, ranging from complete despair to limited optimism. She had no idea how I was doing while I was in the ambulance, so she was more than a bit relieved to see me awake in the ER, realizing I'd arrived safely. My son, Noah, was in Los Angeles, and upon learning what had happened, he was able to make his way to my bedside by the next day. Seeing him at my bedside made me both sad and happy at the same time. I was sad to know that he was upset and worried that I might die. I regretted that he had to see his father in such a condition when I had always been like the Rock of Gibraltar, a pillar of strength for my family. I was happy because I knew he would offer help and strength to his sister and mom.

Once we arrived at Good Samaritan Hospital, the transfer from the ambulance was rough. I remember reminding the person moving me that I was a human being, not just a slab of meat, so could they please be a little bit gentler in their handling of me? Once in the ER, I bypassed the usual check-in procedures, as an acute stroke patient is a true medical emergency and is treated as such. I suppose the personnel transferring me had to balance the necessity for speed with my comfort given that they needed to get me to the ER as quickly as possible. Time to diagnosis and the institution of appropriate treatment is a critical factor in the survival rate following a stroke.

After a cursory examination by the ER physician (during which I was again asked the requisite mental status questions), someone was brought in from neurology to perform a more extensive physical exam and ordered a CAT scan and MRI of my brain. Again, I endured transfers from the ER bed to the radiology table and then to the CAT scan table. The transfers continued to be quite rough, and I repeated my request to handle me a little more gently.

While inside the tube of the MRI machine, I was instructed to remain perfectly still and try not to become claustrophobic, which wasn't easy. The machine makes a pounding noise, which sounds like someone a hitting a metal sheet with a ballpeen hammer over and over for the entire duration of the scan. I was given a button to push if I could not tolerate it, but I knew I had to, so I tried to remain perfectly still and think about absolutely anything else. In order to get through the scan one minute at a time, I listened to music in my head, tried to control my breathing, and counted down in hopes that it would speed up the process. While it seemed an interminable amount of time, the scan was finally completed, and I prepared for another rough transfer back to my hospital bed.

At this point, IVs were started, blood was taken for tests, and an indwelling foley catheter was inserted to monitor my urine output. Multiple physicians came into the room to examine me and—yet again—assess my neurological status. I was eventually informed by the next day that I had suffered a hemorrhagic stroke with quite a large bleed on the right side of my brain.

I was not a candidate for the clot buster since there was no clot. The clot buster therapy is officially referred to as TPA (Tissue Plasminogen Activator). It is a special enzyme that can dissolve a clot—if it's given within a certain timeframe after a stroke caused by a blood clot has occurred. Since I had a bleed, the administration of TPA would only make my condition worse. I was also told that if the bleeding continued, I would have to undergo surgery to stop it. This was a reality I wished to avoid, knowing full well that surgically entering and exiting the brain to tie off a bleeder could cause even more damage to my brain tissue and possibly leave me even more disabled.

The immediate treatment decided upon was IV Mannitol to create a diuresis (increased or excessive production of urine) intended to lower the volume in my vascular system and lessen the pressure in the brain where the blood vessel had burst. While the Mannitol coursed through my veins, I chose to remain perfectly still in my bed, stay calm, and pray to any God who would listen. I had many one-way conversations with God, asking Him to let me live and declaring that, for whatever I had done to deserve this, I was terribly sorry. In addition to prayer, I sent mental messages to the clean-up crew in my body, specifically a special cell called a macrophage, to get up to my brain and begin to clean up the blood and any other damaged tissue there. (Macrophages are highly specialized cells involved in the removal of dying or dead cells and cellular debris.)

As my awareness of my lost freedom continued to heighten, I began to more fully assess the effects of the stroke on my body. My freedom, dignity, and identity as a physician were beginning to leave me. I could not move or in any way use my left arm or leg, and my speech was slurred, but I could see and hear everything going on around me and was able to communicate with my family and the medical staff. I could not walk, turn over in bed, or dress myself. Given that I had a catheter in place, I did not have to worry about getting up to urinate.

It would have been natural for me to feel sorry for myself and wallow in self-pity over what had happened to me, but I knew that approach would not get me better. Thus, I decided that I first had to understand exactly how I had been impacted—both mentally and physically— by the hemorrhagic stroke. I believed that with this knowledge in hand, I'd be able to better understand exactly what I needed to do to get better. A long, uncertain journey of working my way back to me was about to begin! Where it would lead, I didn't know—but I was ready to find out!

I was not allowed to eat or drink anything by mouth for fear of choking for at least two days. The Mannitol infusion can cause dehydration, so I became incredibly thirsty. In fact, my mouth was so parched that it felt as though I had been in the desert for days with nothing to drink. I began begging for a sip of water or even a few ice chips, neither of which I was given despite the many bribes I offered. I offered money, cars, my home, *anything* anyone wanted, as the unbearable thirst was, at that point, the worst result of my stroke! Finally, my daughter was allowed to place a little sponge on the end of a stick typically used for mouth hygiene in my mouth. There was a little moisture in the sponge, and I sucked on it so hard that it came off the stick and she had to reach into my mouth to get it out. We had a good laugh about that, but being thirsty was truly the worst of my suffering post-stroke. It felt like torture, and it was my central complaint to anyone nearby.

I could have only sponge baths for at least the first two weeks, which felt like a lifetime. Fortunately, I am right-handed and could use my right hand to brush my teeth and shave in bed, using a bowl of water and a mirror.

During those initial few days, my wife spoke to the admitting neurologist at Good Sam to inquire about my prognosis. The unfortunate reply was, "Your husband had a stroke, and he is paralyzed." She immediately wondered, "What about all the treatments I've heard of that are available for stroke patients?" and concluded I was in the wrong hospital. The next morning, she asked my attending physicians for their prognosis, wondering if it might be different from that of the neurologist. When they didn't offer much hope either and reinforced that I'd most likely be paralyzed, my family decided I should be transferred. Thus, the next morning I was moved (I'll let you guess how comfortable the ambulance ride was) to the neurology ICU at Stanford Medical Center, where I remained for two weeks undergoing repeat CAT scans, more tests to monitor the bleed (which thankfully stopped, after which point CAT scans occurred far less frequently), intensive physical therapy (PT) for my leg, and occupational therapy (OT) for my arm.

About twenty-four hours after transferring to Stanford, I had another scan to determine the status of the bleed. I continued to do everything I could to remain calm and still while hoping for the best. It's critical to remain absolutely still, as any movement interferes with the scan's usefulness. Staying still with that ballpeen hammer hammering away required great focus on my part; as most people who've undergone this type of scan will concur, the experience isn't pleasant (that's an understatement), and I therefore didn't want to have to undertake it any more frequently than necessary due to not getting a good scan.

I learned that friends from all over the world had been praying for me, and I sincerely hoped that one of them—from any religion whatsoever—had a direct line to God through which He would hear my pleas for the bleeding to stop so I could avoid going under the knife.

The scans finally indicated that the bleed had stopped, and I would not need surgery to stop it. Our prayers had been answered; the Mannitol had done its job! I was informed that a large clot had formed in my brain, which the doctors could see on the CAT scan. Receiving this result seemed to take forever, but I subsequently learned that everything related to having had a stroke would take more time than I wanted, so I'd better learn some patience and slow down when it came to wanting everything immediately and being inherently quite impulsive.

We were told that the bleed would slowly resolve on its

own, and it was time to ascertain my physical and cognitive limitations in order to create and implement a treatment plan so I could begin the process of regaining as much of the freedom I had lost as possible.

A repeat assessment of my ability to swallow led to a decision to gradually advance my orally ingested diet from nothing to soft food to semi-solid food to solid food. I must say, the initial soft diet had the look and taste of library paste and was absolutely disgusting. I tolerated it well without choking, so I progressed to semi-solid food. It wasn't until I was finally given solid food that I was able to appreciate the culinary delights that are produced in a hospital kitchen. Thankfully, my son brought me a fast-food burger and fries, which were delightful and cause for a mini celebration.

With the Mannitol infusion complete, a regular (sugar-water) IV helped reverse my dehydration and craving for liquids. Interestingly, I developed a craving for Doritos chips and the Wendy's Frosty (half vanilla, half chocolate). Of course, once a lover of a half-and-half Wendy's Frosty, always a lover, and I still enjoy Doritos (though my taste buds have expanded to appreciate the new, spicier versions).

When I finally had to poop (which took about a week given that I wasn't eating very much), I struggled with a bed pan. The entire process was quite difficult and most unpleasant. One time, the staff used a cradle to lift me from my bed and place me on a toilet, which I proceeded to clog when one of my socks fell in. Water flowed all over the bathroom floor, causing a plumbing emergency in Stanford hospital. It was like a scene out of the movie "Keystone Cops"!

While I'm not sure whether this event was the primary impetus for my transfer from Stanford to another inpatient facility a few days later, I was informed that I had survived my acute, post-stroke period and was now in need of longer-term inpatient PT, OT, and speech therapy, none of which was offered at Stanford. Imagine our surprise at this news. How could a world-class medical center like Stanford not offer these kinds of services for stroke/TBI survivors?

We were given a basic list of inpatient rehab facilities in the South Bay area without any accompanying guidance or direction, so my wife and daughter personally visited every single facility on the list. The one that had the most activity and staff present (even though it was Saturday), as well as the opportunity for me to have my own room was Santa Clara Valley Medical Center. Upon further research, we discovered that it had a well-equipped rehab facility and an excellent reputation. So, it was "VMC, here I come!" for my next six weeks of my recovery.

I recommend strongly that the patient's family visits these facilities before making a selection, as they are not equal in what they provide. My wife and daughter prioritized the following qualities as they assessed our options:

- A facility associated with a hospital so that physicians would be available at all times to address any new issues that might arise
- A robust rehab unit that provided physical,

occupational, and speech therapy services
- Lots of visible activity in the rehab unit seven days a week
- Adequate nursing staff to manage the patient load

Once admitted to VMC, I was initially greeted by Dr. Duong, a physical rehab physician in charge of their inpatient rehab service. She and I discussed my case in great detail, physician to physician, and Dr. Duong would continue to be wonderful, skillful, and extremely caring during the next period of my recovery.

During my time in the rehab facility, I had lots of time to think about what had happened to me, and the first question that occurred was, not surprisingly, *WHY?* My blood pressure had been under control for years, as had my cholesterol. I did not have any heart irregularities or underlying tendency for vascular malformations in my brain. So *why* did I have a bleed? No one could answer that question, but I quickly came to the realization there was no answer. My time and energy would be better spent understanding my deficits and learning what I had to do in order to return (as much as possible) to my pre-stroke status and go home. My advice to other survivors is not to focus on the "why" but to simply get on with their recovery program as soon as possible!

Every night, I prayed to God to let me heal and wake up the next morning in better shape than I was the night before. If I had done something wrong, I asked God for forgiveness and vowed that I would never make the same mistake again. Needless to say, intensive prayer was not the sole answer. There was no magic bullet or medicine or deal to be made that would, on its own, make me better. Each day I woke up I believed to be a gift, I was ready once again to do battle in my recovery to get better and return home.

After discussing my situation with my new therapists at VMC, what was abundantly clear was that the solution required that I commit to working hard in my therapy sessions so that I could begin to regain some use in my left arm and leg. How much improvement I would be able to make would be determined over time, and there were no overnight miracles to be expected. Every survivor is different with respect to their deficit and the timeframe in which they will see improvement. Thus, no prescribed generalizations on progress are possible. This is a critical concept to accept because what survivors want to immediately know is how long it will take to get better. Unfortunately, there is no definitive answer to this question. In fact, I have met survivors who are *still* improving, even twenty years post-stroke.

With my therapists, I committed to the following:

EARLY COMMITMENTS

1. I would be the hardest working therapy patient they ever had seen.

2. I would adopt the attitude to never, ever, *ever* give up.

3. I would do everything my therapists asked me to do without fear.

4. I would work to exhaustion if necessary; there was plenty of time to rest.

5. I would read every book by other stroke survivors to identify any insights that could speed up or otherwise aid my recovery.

6. When in a therapy session, I would always do one more of whatever they asked me to do. I called it "One more for good luck."

7. I would set realistic, achievable goals with my therapists and strive to attain them.

8. I would investigate all treatments for stroke patients (that were not dangerous) that might help me, including hyperbaric oxygen, stem cells, various braces to facilitate walking and use of my hand, acupuncture, and Botox for spasticity.

These eight declarations defined my attitude at this stage of my recovery as I committed to regaining my freedom and my physical capabilities as much as possible.

I made sure to celebrate even the "small" achievements. Baby steps/small goals are very important in achieving and defining progress, and they included doing something one day that I could not do the day before. That small win motivated me to work even harder and with more determination not to let the stroke win. In my case, some of my small wins included the ability to speak more quickly in a short period of time, the ability to read and comprehend, and the ability to use a wheelchair without crashing into walls.

I vowed to win with hard work. I vowed not to be defeated by the stroke nor to let the stroke determine who I would be going forward. That piece was key in defining the person I would be post-stroke, as life will never be the same for me or for my family. It's important that I include my family here and that each stroke survivor does the same, because an important concept for the patient, their family, and all others instrumental in their life to acknowledge is that the stroke did not just happen to the patient. Stroke is the leading cause of disability in the world today. However, no one is every truly prepared for the life-changing aftermath of suffering a stroke. The trauma of a stroke is not mutually exclusive to the patient; it significantly affects the entire family.

CHAPTER TWO

Regaining Freedom and Independence

STROKE FACT

Following any type of stroke, it is well known (and part of making the diagnosis of a stroke) that the patient is immediately unable to do certain things such as speak clearly, walk, or move their arms or legs, which requires them to need assistance as their previous ability to care for themselves is not possible until some degree of recovery occurs.

Soon after having a stroke, the patient is forced to come to terms with what they can and cannot do. I referred to this process as "losing my freedom and independence," as I needed help to get dressed, wash up, and use the bathroom; cut up my food; have someone bring me items that weren't within easy reach; turn over in bed; and whatever else could not be accomplished with the use of only one arm.

Falling is a universal fear that stroke and TBI patients share as they begin taking their first steps while in physical therapy. After being on bedrest or confined to a wheelchair for varying lengths of time, the desire is to be back on one's feet and begin to re-learn to walk. Balance is a major issue central to one's ability to stand and walk, which contributes to the fear of falling. To date, I have fallen fourteen times since my stroke, and I'm happy to report that my years as a horseman served me well in more ways than I could have imagined, having been bucked off a number of horses and therefore learned how to shoulder-roll—similar to landing with a parachute—in order to avoid serious injury.

Each time I fell, it was due to a different "mistake," such as miscalculating my next step or otherwise forgetting to properly calculate my next move while getting from Point A to Point B. To fall as a result of trying to relearn to walk is a risk the patient must assume. However, to fall again after making the same mistake suggests that one didn't learn from his previous error. Thus, if one falls again, it should be for a new reason or mistake—one that can be subsequently corrected! To that end, I am happy to report that each of my fourteen falls was for a different reason.

My first fall occurred while I was sitting on the edge of the bed shortly after returning home. I was reaching for something on the bedside table. Whatever I was reaching for was just a bit out of reach, and I slipped off the bed and onto the floor. I realized I had misjudged the distance and should have asked for help, but I was too stubborn and suffered the consequence: my first fall.

After a bit of crying from surprise and disappointment—not from any injury sustained—Lana comforted me and asked what I was going to do next. I told her I was going to use the techniques I'd learned from my therapists to get up and back into bed. Actually, first I said, "I'm getting back in bed, and I'm never getting out again." (Despite that declaration, the next morning I indeed got up in order to continue my rehab.)

I'd learned that after a fall, I was to crawl over to something sturdy like a chair or a counter and work to get my leg (the one with the AFO brace on it) under me. At that point, I would reach up to the chair or counter and push off my good right leg in order to stand up on both feet. If someone is present, they can assist me in this adventure, which makes it much easier. However, it is critical to be able to get up on your own, as at least one fall is more than likely to occur when you are alone.

Another time, I caught the toe of my shoe on a crack in the sidewalk, and I occasionally lost my balance climbing stairs that didn't have a railing. The most embarrassing "mistake" I made was when Lana was helping me go down the walkway on the side of our house while I was in a wheelchair. The steep incline caused her to lose her grip on the chair, and both of us fell down—while I was still in the wheelchair! We both laughed and cried before going to the garage, where I could climb the stairs to the first floor using the handrail.

As I reached the top step, I again fell forward while trying to step onto the landing. I hit my head on the wall, but not terribly hard. That made for two falls in one day! Each of these falls could have been avoided had I taken the time to understand the inherent risks and what I could (and should) have done to mitigate them. As I incorporated that level of attention into my walking, the number of falls lessened, and there was more time between them. Thankfully, nothing but my pride was hurt as a result of my falls, and they each provided another opportunity to acknowledge the reality of my new limitations and commit to being more careful in the future. I learned that when attempting something new, I had to first assess in detail what I was attempting and where the risks were so I could take action to mitigate another fall.

I remind other stroke survivors that falls will happen as we strive to take chances in order to regain our lost freedom, but I also encourage them not to be afraid of falling. If and when you do fall, simply do a shoulder roll, as if you were landing from a parachute jump or falling off a bucking horse (which, as I mentioned, I had a lot of experience with. I've ridden horses since I was very young) and be sure to ask your physical therapist to show you how to get up should you happen to fall.

CHAPTER THREE

Depression

STROKE MYTH

Associated depression is not worth treating.

D espite how committed I was to staying focused on positivity, depression soon made an appearance soon after moving to VMC and beginning my active phase of rehabilitation. I was considered to have a Type-A personality pre-stroke, and suddenly the rug had been pulled out from under me, rendering me largely helpless. This was devastating. So devastating, in fact, that it led to bouts of uncontrollable crying—many "blue moments." I was clearly on an emotional roller coaster, which was totally not me—the stoic, macho physician and CEO of a company who had always been able to easily control his inner feelings. I felt emotionally naked! These feelings began to occur frequently while doing my rehab at VMC as the reality of the tough road ahead became quite apparent. I recognized that there would be no easy win in this battle. My worst moments occurred when I was alone and exhausted from therapy sessions.

Let's be honest, who wouldn't be depressed by such a sudden loss of freedom and dignity? My strong personality—both as a physician with the power to heal others and as a businessman successful in leading R&D and acting as CEO of a company—delayed my willingness to admit my depression and take prescribed medication to minimize it.

I quickly learned that emotional lability (or volatility) is a common post-stroke occurrence, and crying was okay because it was a part of my healing. I continued to focus on what I could do, not on what I couldn't do, and this helped me maintain my focus on working hard to regain my freedom.

Nighttime might be considered the worst period of the day for a stroke patient, as loneliness envelops you like a bound-up mummy! You are left alone with your thoughts and listening to your breathing pattern and heartbeat until sleep finally and kindly takes its hold and allows you some rest and a bit of time to perhaps dream about more pleasant thoughts. Listening to the PA system announce that patients were in trouble or hearing the arrival of a helicopter were terribly distracting occurrences that could trigger depression, knowing another patient in trouble was arriving.

One solution we devised to help me feel a bit better during my in-patient recovery period revolved around my wife's colorful scarves. Each night as Lana left VMC, I enjoyed smelling her perfume during our hug goodnight. I asked her, "Why don't you leave me your scarf sprayed with your perfume, and I can wrap it around my pillow and smell it all night long while I try to sleep alone here at the hospital." This became a much-anticipated ritual, and I am convinced it facilitated my ability to get a good night's sleep and feel less alone. Some gave me strange looks when they learned what I was doing, but I couldn't have cared less. One night, however, probably from moving my head a lot and sweating, the color from the scarf transferred to my hair. When my wife and daughter arrived the next morning and entered my room, they both began to laugh. I looked like Rainbow Man with multiple colors in my hair. (Rainbow Man was a fixture at NBA games, sporting a rainbow-colored Afro wig while holding signs with religious messages for all to see.) It took a few shampoos to get the colors out of my hair, and from then on, all the scarves Lana left me were colorless so I would not have any more color changes to my hair in the morning.

Everyone thought that the changing hair color incident was hilarious, to which I said, "I'm glad you're enjoying this so much at my expense!" But when I looked in the mirror, I had to admit it was pretty funny, Nevertheless, I did not enjoy being the butt of jokes considering the position I was in! That being said, maintaining a sense of humor during this time was very helpful to me. Fortunately, having an inherently good sense of humor served me well.

In hindsight, resistance both to the depression itself and to a willingness to consider medication to help treat it was a clear mistake on my part. I advise new stroke patients that it is okay to cry. I still do occasionally, even eleven years later. Crying is part of the healing process. I still cry occasionally, even eleven years later. The emotional rollercoaster returns every so often, sometimes totally unexpectedly, and I can't help myself from succumbing to shedding some tears, mainly out of frustration for how long it sometimes takes to get even a little better and how tired and depressed I feel, trapped in my present physical condition. Everything I want to do requires that I expend so much effort! Yet I have to remind myself of the progress I have made and what I can do rather than how difficult some things still are for me.

I feel like a fighter who keeps getting knocked down but must rally, get up off the canvas, and get back in the fight. In my case, the fight is getting back into the struggle of my recovery program. I tell myself to turn all the energy expended on crying and feeling upset into working more on my recovery program with my therapists and caregivers.

My family was quite upset each time they witnessed me crying; it was an unusual sight for them. Fortunately, they are all strong individuals, and in addition to hugging me and telling me how much better I was doing, they would also hug each other and support each other in committing as a group to helping me get through the low moments and assisting in my recovery program. They could not have been more supportive, and thus, whenever I would experience a low moment, I would think about how much my family wanted me back. This motivated me to snap out of a "blue moment" and get back to my program. Anti-depressant medication helped to keep the "blue moments" away for long periods of time, for which I was thankful.

Please consider discussing the option of medicating your depression with your medical provider so that you can focus on your recovery. I advise family members that if their loved one is crying, simply hug them. Tell them you love them and that it is okay to cry and get it out of their system. Then, re-focus their energy on getting back in the game of working harder to improve.

CHAPTER FOUR

The Birth of Dr. K

STROKE FACT

Following a stroke or brain injury, the patient may feel as though life (as they lived it previously) is over, especially when they believe their physical limitations are permanent. This is the time when a discussion needs to happen surrounding the fact that they can reverse some of their new limitations if they are ready to engage in a comprehensive rehabilitation program. This is the first step in beginning to define who they will be following the stroke, what I refer to as "the new you." Each patient has to define who and what they want to be in the future instead of wallowing in self-pity and giving up.

At VMC, the staff was often confused about how to refer to me, knowing I was a physician. Calling me "Dr. Krochmal" was difficult because it's not the easiest name to pronounce. Therefore, to make things easier for everyone, my alter ego emerged, and I became "Dr. K."

I even had a sign on the wall in my room that read "Please call me Dr. K," which was well received by everyone, and I was happily defining the new Dr. K.

As Dr. K, I became known for the statements "One more for good luck," "I refuse to let the stroke win," and "Never, never, ever give up." I apparently uttered each of them frequently. This period of time was when I began to define myself anew. I was becoming more open-minded, more outgoing, less judgmental, more patient, less demanding, and less impulsive. This shift was readily noticed by my family, who was used to me being exactly the opposite!

The physician/helper in me also began to re-emerge, and along with a fellow stroke survivor named Nathan Daniel, I created the website www.postroke.com while at VMC. Through this website, we told our stories and provided what we hoped would be useful information for other new survivors.

During this time, I was also actively engaged in physical, occupational, and speech therapy, realizing that success in those areas would allow me to return home sooner than later. Additionally, I took part in vocational therapy once a week with other patients, through which we engaged in simple activities such as tie-dying T-shirts, painting, playing games, and even taking a road trip to Barnes and Noble, which marked my first trip out of the hospital and back out into the real world. I initially thought that these kinds of activities were "below" me and childish. After all, I was a physician! But I came to understand their helpful role in my recovery as well as the benefits of the camaraderie that developed between patients, which carried over into our therapy sessions. We frequently cheered each other on and yelled out encouragement to each other.

I vividly remember watching my new comrades attempt something difficult during their therapy session. I also recall telling a patient who was screaming in pain during therapy that screaming is not allowed. There is no screaming, as it upsets other patients who are trying to do their best in therapy and don't want the distraction that screaming causes. In response, the screamer stopped, and the therapists had a good chuckle at my compassionately honest approach.

Before long, I discovered that even though I had previously perceived myself as an outgoing, engaging extrovert, I was clearly going to take my outgoing nature to a new level. I proactively said hello to strangers; made small talk more readily; and engaged more often with others in wheelchairs to compare experiences, inquire as to their progress, and encourage them to work hard and never give up. When other patients were struggling a bit or crying out in pain, I tried to console them and encourage them to take the energy involved in crying and apply it instead to the exercises they were doing to get better. It often seemed to help, and their therapists seemed most appreciative of my unsolicited intervention.

I came to terms with my loss of freedom and dignity by realizing I had no other choice. My family wanted to help me, and they also wanted me to be able to ask them for help. As I accepted our new reality, each family member took on certain tasks as assigned. For example, my daughter was in charge of my laptop and email and took responsibility for handling my work-related duties. She was also responsible for scheduling visits from friends, which had to be limited because they exhausted me due to the effort required to focus and engage in conversation. I never realized how tiring such visits could be. All visitors were forewarned that my attention span was limited, and their visit would therefore be limited as a result. I was grateful that everyone was very respectful of this and left promptly when I said I was tired and needed to rest.

My wife, son, and daughter all helped me with meals, dressing, and personal hygiene, which was the most difficult aspect of help to accept. I had changed their diapers as babies, but now they had to help me clean up after a bowel movement. No fun! My son stayed with me in my room almost every night to ensure that if I needed something, he could take care of it. When my son needed a break, my daughter stayed with me. My son brought me food I craved from time to time (starting with that first hamburger and fries I spoke of earlier), and my family got me a tablet so I could listen to music and stay current with the news. My wife read the paper to me every day.

Each family member had to learn how to safely help me transfer from bed to wheelchair and demonstrate their proficiency in this task to my therapists before I could be sent home. I believed that my ability to make safe transfers was key to returning home, so it became a main focus. The most important step in becoming more independent was learning how to transfer from the bed to a wheelchair. Once this skill was mastered, I was able to transfer to the exercise table for therapy, the commode (no more bed pan), the shower bench, and even into a car. I continued to be able to access more and more freedom, which was invigorating!

CHAPTER FIVE

Find Humor in the Mundane

STROKE FACT

Laughter in and of itself can be healing and has been recognized for many years as a healing modality that provides relief from stress associated with many serious illnesses.

According to the Mayo clinic, "A good sense of humor can't cure all ailments, but data is mounting about the positive things laughter can do."

Because laughter can induce extremely positive physical and emotional changes in the body, a stroke survivor is a perfect candidate to benefit from laughter. The key is to find laughter available in one's environment (i.e., the hospital). By being extra observant, it's not hard to find a variety of funny things occurring during the rehab stage of recovery. In addition, watching funny movies (I'll list my favorites in the Appendix) made me laugh, and finding funny shows to watch on my tablet was also a great source of entertainment for me.

While at both Stanford and VMC, I had a seemingly never-ending stream of staff physicians, residents, and medical students flowing in and out of my room, conducting repeat neurological exams. I did not mind this at all. As a physician, I understood the value of this teaching opportunity, and I instructed each practitioner that they were welcome to examine me, however they could not leave any more of me uncovered than they had found upon arrival! Saying this to the young doctors caused a bit of laughter for everyone, given the obvious range of what I'd dare to say to them!

They poked me all over with a sharp pin to track where I noticed feeling, which continued to be diminished on my impacted left arm and leg. Otherwise, I felt every pinprick, and they each hurt! When asked if I felt anything sharp, I'd respond, "I had a stroke, but I am not dead!" Of course, everyone (including me) laughed.

I began to spend more time with other patients on the ward at meals as well as outside on a patio where I was able to enjoy the fresh air and see the blue sky, trees, birds, and squirrels. It made me feel alive, and I knew I had to continue my hard work so I could go home. I really wanted my life back! I also began to look at the other stroke patients as my brothers and sisters, as we were all in the same boat, worried about our futures and our ability to get better.

To help me focus on pushing forward, I created a "wall of love" in my room where get-well cards and other messages were posted, along with a list of the PT and OT goals I had to achieve before I could go home. This allowed me to read them upon awakening each morning and retiring at night, and it kept my attention to my goals sharp, reinforced my commitment, and renewed my commitment to achieving them.

When my OT determined I was ready to take a shower (after I had mastered safe transfers), I was so happy. I'd missed taking showers since suffering my stroke. Hygiene had been maintained with sponge baths which got me clean but also reminded me of my loss of dignity, given that I was dependent upon others to be washed and dried. I looked forward to my first real shower, accompanied by my occupational therapist, Hubert, who would assist me. Hubert told me not to get him wet, and I told him I could not promise him that. Of course, I made sure to spray him, causing a good laugh that he and I shared!

I had my own shampoo and soap from home and used my wheelchair to get into a special shower where I transferred myself to a shower bench and used a handheld shower to get wet. With my right hand, I was able to shampoo my hair and wash most of my body with a washcloth. It is hard to convey how great the warm water felt running over my head and body as I rinsed. I hand plenty of towels with which to dry, and then I was back in my wheelchair, heading back to my room. I was so happy that I screamed out loud to anyone nearby, "I feel like a new man!" My family was awaiting me, and after transferring back into bed, they helped me dress for the day. They were so happy because I finally had a happy smile on my face. Needless to say, I looked forward to my shower every few days.

I received a nightly injection into my abdomen to prevent my blood from forming clots, as I was not ambulating very much. The injection hurt like hell, so I always told the nurse just before she administered it, "Aim twice, poke once, because this hurts!" The nurse always laughed with me. I counted down the shots to my last one, which served as another sign that I was getting closer to discharge.

Some of my meals at VMC were okay, but truthfully, most were horrible. My daughter got so upset with what my dinner looked like one night that she threw my entire tray into the garbage. We had noticed that in the yard in front of the hospital, the population of black squirrels was going down, and that prompted me to inquire as to whether I was eating squirrel for some meals. Before long, I was able to negotiate with my doctor and the nutritionist to have bacon with my breakfast and a Ball Park hot dog for lunch. Both were really good! Another small win for me, the patient!

Upon learning that I was a dermatologist, nurses and aides would pop into my room and ask me to look at something on their skin. Here I was, trying to recover from a stroke, but that did not stop anybody from asking these questions! I told them what I could when it came to how to treat their problem, and if it was something that required further treatment, I referred them to a colleague. I was always happy to help anyone because they were all helping me, which I so deeply appreciated. This minor imposition on my expertise gave me a smile and made me chuckle, considering the circumstances.

Once I was able to use a bedside commode for bowel movements, I had to have several aids help transfer me from the bed to the commode. Those who helped me were referred to by me as My All-Commode Team to bring a little levity to the execution of an unpleasant but necessary bodily function. I submitted the names of my All-Commode team on a card that would ensure special recognition for them in a future staff meeting. I thoroughly enjoyed being a bit of a wise guy and doing things just for a laugh.

Other things I did to keep my sense of humor and joy intact included passing the time by listening to music and watching funny movies on my iPad. My son, Noah, suggested a number of movies to me, including "Dude, Where's my Car?", "Planes, Trains and Automobiles," and "Uncle Buck."

Some of my favorite songs when it came to cheering me up included "I'm Free" by The Who and "Keep on Pushing" by The Impressions. I sang these songs to myself in my head as I do not have a singer's voice. My speech therapists recommended several brain games that I enjoyed as well, including Lumosity (this was my favorite), BrainHG, Elevate, and My Brain Trainer. The brain games were fun, as you could monitor your progress, proving once again that there were lots of small gains available to be achieved, which was quite motivating to me.

It's so important for the stroke survivor's emotional and physical recovery that they identify humorous moments during their recovery, as doing so provides a sign to all that they still possess a sense of humor. This knowledge is extremely reassuring to families, loved ones, and caregivers/therapists. Even though stroke recovery is a difficult and frustrating road, one can still find lighter moments and humorous instances if only he takes a moment to look for them.

CHAPTER SIX

The Therapist Ticket

STROKE FACT

Your therapists often hold the "You Can Go Home Now" ticket, so learning to work with them effectively is critical.

It soon became apparent by watching them with other patients that they had a very difficult job indeed. I wondered how they managed to wake up each morning feeling energized to come to work and do their best to help depressed stroke survivors work to get better and realized part of it likely involved *knowing* that they were making a difference. Therefore, I knew that I had to show them that what they did for me each day was truly helping me. I had to demonstrate progress so they would be motivated to come back to work each day to assist me and to give me their best. When I discussed my thoughts on all of this with them, they agreed, and this mutual understanding was a very important bonding concept for both patient and therapist.

Stroke patients often have to employ other muscles and nerve pathways to regain use of their arms and legs, and accomplishing this requires many repetitions of the same exercise or movement. The process of the brain utilizing alternate neural connections is referred to as "neuroplasticity." With this in mind, whatever number of repetitions of an exercise I was asked to do, I always said at the end that I wanted to do one more for good luck, and my therapists were very happy to see me do it. I was once asked why I had that approach, and I responded that if I did one more every time, after a year I may have done hundreds more than called for, and this might hasten my recovery. It was all about reps, reps, and more reps to foster neuroplasticity, which is the ability to use undamaged areas of the brain to send neuromuscular signals to muscle groups to contract or relax. This is a critical component of the recovery process for both stroke and TBI survivors to understand.

The concept of neuroplasticity should be explained to every survivor, their family members, and their caregivers, as it helps them better understand why repetition in therapy sessions (and also while doing exercises at home) is so important in obtaining and maintaining improvement.

Thinking back on my rehab program, I must say that I was surprised by the degree of effort and repetition required to make tangible progress, not to mention the degree of commitment and determination necessary to stay with the program and not give up out of frustration and slower-than-desired improvement. Most days, it was a challenge to muster the strength and determination required to get through another day of therapy and living with my new physical limitations.

Nevertheless, therapy is your only real ticket to going home and continuing your life, albeit in a newly altered fashion. Having another chance to continue your life is the real gift of a rehab program. The harder you work, the better you do. So get with it!

Oftentimes in therapy, the patient is requested to do something that seems difficult, risky, or dangerous—or all three. I readily accepted the challenge and commented to my therapists that I relied on them to give me the courage and confidence to try if they thought I was ready. Invariably, I was able to do what I was asked to do. For example, walk without a cane (which was very scary, but it was a great accomplishment and another major milestone achieved)! All of my therapists gave me the confidence and courage necessary to try to do things that, at first glance, seemed risky. But I had trained hard for that challenge, and I always accomplished what they asked me to do. I had to move beyond my comfort zone many times, but by doing so, I became even more motivated to keep going!

In retrospect, the therapist was right if she thought I was ready to do something a bit risky. I was so grateful that they gave me the courage and confidence to try, and we both celebrated when I accomplished the task!

As I reflect on my time with my various therapists, it is obvious there were some with whom I was more in sync than others. My present PT and OT know me so well (and vice versa) that I have told them that they play my body like a piano. Plus, they have hands of steel, which is awfully reassuring when doing something I consider risky. With just the slightest touch or nudge, I knew exactly what they wanted me to do, which usually involves correcting something during an exercise. Don't be afraid to occasionally change therapists until you find one with whom you really are comfortable, who understands your needs and is committed to helping you make the progress you seek.

I counsel other stroke patients to not be afraid when asked by their therapists to do something. They are there to give you the courage and confidence you need to try! My progress undeniably motivated my therapists to give me *their* best each and every day. I wanted them to give me their best, so it was only fair that I gave them *my* best during therapy sessions. I'd never been a slacker, and I wasn't about to start now! I give thanks to God almighty for providing me with this character trait.

CHAPTER SEVEN

Preparing to Go Home

STROKE FACT

Going home is not a simple process. Most determined stroke and TBI patients focus on learning about the "going home" process early on in their recovery phase. It's important to understand what skills you must be able to demonstrate before discharge, what modifications need to be made to your living quarters, how you will continue your rehab program, and what equipment is needed at home. Many of the answers can be provided by your therapists and/or the social services representative assigned to you.

A bout two weeks prior to my discharge home from VMC (I was a patient there for approximately eight weeks), my physical and occupational therapist accompanied us for a required visit to my home to assess whether any physical modifications would be necessary to support my return. As I had been taught how to transfer from the bed to a wheelchair and then again to a treatment table, transferring from the wheelchair to a seat in my car was easy. I mastered that skill, knowing it was critical for the future I desired.

Riding home in the car was exhilarating. Just to see the world again—the world that I had so dearly missed those past few months—was an indescribable feeling. I opened the window to enjoy the breeze and fresh air while listening to the sounds of the city that I had missed so much during my confinement.

In order for me to get inside my home, two strong men picked me up in my wheelchair and carried me up the dozen or so front steps into the house. Even though it was a very brief visit, I was so happy to see my home and everything inside that I had missed. We quickly realized that more railings were needed along the stairway from the garage to the first floor of the house, as well as from the first floor to our bedroom. We also needed a walkway around the house for wheelchair access and a ramp built over the stairs so I could enter the house through the backdoor. I would need a bed in our family room where we would sleep, as I was not yet able to climb the stairs to our bedroom. Luckily, there was a bathroom nearby the family room with a shower I could use. In addition to a wheelchair, a transfer chair and bedside commode were needed. Thanks to my family, acquiring or building all of this was somehow accomplished in the two weeks prior to my discharge.

Find an experienced contractor to do any necessary work. Ask your therapists or other stroke survivors for recommendations. When interviewing a contractor, be sure to ask if they have the relevant, requisite experience in getting a home ready for wheelchair access and to allow for easy navigating once the survivor is inside. Don't forget to check into modifications needed in the bathroom and shower too. It's extremely important to ensure that these two areas are as safe as possible.

During my inpatient treatment (as well as once I returned home), there were several devices that I was able to utilize when it came to assisting with walking or hand function. It's important to discuss these devices with your own therapist, as they can recommend which might be best for your particular situation. Some of the devices I was able to try included:

Bioness
I used the hand model, and it did stimulate my hand to open. Important to note is the fact that it requires ongoing support and adjustment by a Bioness technician. The foot drop device did not help in my case.

Walk-Aide
Unfortunately, neither the hand or foot device gave me any benefit, but it's a respected option so check with your therapist to see if it might be a good one for you to try.

Saebo
I used and liked the Saebo-stretch brace. It helped with the stiff tone in my hand. The Saebo glove was also helpful in

opening my fingers allowing me to grip objects.

The following equipment was incredibly useful (if not mandatory) and can be obtained from a general equipment supplier for handicapped individuals:

- Bedside commode
- Wheelchair
- Transport chair
- Sliding shower bench with a cutout for a good booty wash
- Traveling shower bench

CHAPTER EIGHT

Rehab Fatigue

STROKE MYTH

Most improvement occurs within first six months.

R ehab fatigue is a term I coined to explain a common phenomenon experienced by many of the stroke and TBI survivors I have spoken to, and one I experienced as well. Not surprisingly, the phenomenon has also been confirmed by many therapists.

Oftentimes, at some point during the first two years following the stroke or injury (and even beyond that timeframe), the survivor loses interest in their recovery process and becomes bored with their therapy routine. This may occur out of frustration due to the slow rate of improvement, pain experienced during therapy and exercise, or a belief in the false dogma that all major benefits occur by six months post stroke/injury. The survivor loses interest and their commitment wanes when it comes to the energy and effort required during therapy and exercise. This is a worrisome problem, and it is one that is not only noticed by the survivor but also by the family, caregivers, and therapists.

I began to experience a bit of rehab fatigue while at VMC, primarily from being so tired from the effort expended in my therapy sessions. My primary approach to addressing this was to sleep more at night and take a nap after my therapy, which really helped. Once I was home and undergoing outpatient PT and OT, the fatigue began to occur as a result of having these sessions back-to-back or having too many in a week. We identified these as scheduling issues that were easily resolved by no longer scheduling PT and OT back-to-back and never more than once a week for each one. In addition, my goals were reassessed, as noted in my suggestions below.

The question quickly becomes: What can one do to regain their motivation and commitment to continue working hard on their recovery in order to continue to improve?

Suggestions for Regaining Motivation

- Take a break from therapy/exercising for a few days or weeks and do something that you enjoy instead. This break should not be too long, as it can be a slippery slope when it comes to benefits gained quickly being lost. Neuroplasticity is tough to regain, so you don't want to lose any advances you have gained in this respect.

- Remember what you can do rather than dwell on what you can't do.
- Treat any concomitant depression that could be contributing to the lack of interest in the recovery effort.
- Discuss how you feel with your therapists so that you can work together to recast your goals into perhaps fewer and smaller incremental goals that are easier to achieve and acknowledge.
- Recast your home exercise program into a manageable schedule, alternating exercise programs to add variety. Don't do the same program every day!
- Set a date for returning to PT and OT therapy.
- Speak with survivors who continue to improve many months or even years following their stroke/injury in order to remind yourself that improvement can continue to occur even many years later.
- Keep in mind that every patient is different in their response to therapy. Exercise and repetition are required—sometimes thousands of times—to obtain neuroplasticity, which is the ability of the brain to find new neural connections to carry messages to muscles to relax and contract when nerves were damaged from the stroke or injury. Repetition of an exercise is critical for neuroplasticity to occur.
- Remember, no work, no gain.
- Recommit to work hard, and never, ever give up!
- Be mindful and even suspicious of quick fixes, cures, and treatments offered on the Internet, as they are mainly expensive scams that may be risky and often

do not delivery what is promised. Discuss them with your physicians, therapists, and rehab physicians before taking part in a treatment you may later regret! Unfortunately, there exist deranged individuals who prey on the suffering of stroke and TBI patients and will attempt to take advantage of your position.

CHAPTER NINE

Keeping a Positive Attitude

STROKE FACT

Staying positive following a stroke or TBI is critically important not only for the survivor but also for the family, caregivers, therapists, nurses, and physicians who interact with the survivor.

As I progressed with my therapy sessions, I was frequently asked, "How are you doing?" My standard response was, "Better than yesterday, but not as good as tomorrow," which was totally consistent with my intention to beat this stroke and my never-give-up attitude. Most people who heard my response smiled and agreed, and I could sense that other stroke patients were motivated by my response, which was a nice feeling.

An important outcome from interactions with other stroke survivors at VMC was the appreciation that a stroke was the great equalizer. For those who had unfortunately experienced one, it happened regardless of age, race, skin color, sex, income, or profession. It happened regardless of anything other than known preexisting conditions that had not been identified or treated, such as high blood pressure, high cholesterol, cardiac arrhythmias, or a genetic predisposition to vascular malformations in the brain.

As a physician, I initially thought, "This can't be happening to me." I was quite healthy, active, a nonsmoker, and not a heavy drinker. So how could this happen to me? But it did! I felt, as did others, that the stroke had me sitting in the bottom of the shit bucket, scraping and clawing to get out. Through daily therapy, I could occasionally grip the edge of the bucket just enough to hoist myself up and peer out to see the real world around me. It was beautiful, and I wanted so badly to return to it. So, whatever it would take, I would do it.

This determination was reinforced in one session of physical therapy, before which I had been fitted with an AFO brace for my left ankle and foot. The brace was intended to stabilize my left ankle when I stood up and protect it when I attempted to walk. My lower left leg, ankle, and foot muscles had undergone paresis from the stroke, which is essentially muscle weakness with the inability to walk. At the same time, I had severe tone (tightness) in the muscles of my ankle and foot, which negatively impacted my ability to walk. The brace protected my ankle from further damage, especially from twisting and fracturing when taking my first steps.

My physical therapist at VMC, Sonia (who was fantastic), asked me one day after a few weeks of PT if I was ready to try to take a few steps. I said, "If you think I have progressed sufficiently enough in my recovery that I am ready to try, then hell yes, let's do it!" With a very strong aide behind me, Sonia to my left side, and my right hand holding onto a railing along the wall, I rose out of my wheelchair like a phoenix rising from the ashes. When I just stood and looked around me, Sonia was worried and asked why I had stopped. I replied that I was enjoying the view from a standing position; it was so beautiful compared to what I'd seen the past weeks lying flat in bed, mainly staring at the ceiling.

It is so important to communicate well and frequently with your therapist so that they know how you are feeling. Sonia understood what I was experiencing and did not push me to start walking until I was ready. She appreciated that a standing view for a survivor who had been confined to a bed or wheelchair for weeks was an important thing to behold for a few minutes!

I then took a few steps, and the view continued to change as I passed other patients and therapists in the hallway. I experienced such exhilaration at that moment that I cried tears of happiness and thankfulness, referred to as "happy tears," in stark contrast compared to the tears I shed during "blue moments." This was my first experience crying happy tears in celebration of what I had accomplished for the first time since suffering the stroke. It made me believe I could win the battle to recover. Fortunately, I had only been cognitively compromised for a short time with slurred speech and left-sided neglect, because my stroke occurred on the right side of my brain. Thankfully, I never lost my memory or ability to understand, solve puzzles, think abstractly, or read. In that regard, I had been blessed.

When I returned to my room after that first walking session, my family embraced me. Seeing my tears, they thought I was upset, so I introduced them to this new concept of me crying happy tears when something good happened!

Prior to my departure from VMC, which had been my home for the previous two months, Dr. Duong mentioned to me that VMC wanted to establish an outpatient Stroke Survivors group, and she asked if I would agree to lead it. After discussed this with my wife (the commitment would be to lead 90-minute-long monthly meetings), I agreed, provided the group could be chaired by both my wife and me. I felt this leadership approach would be more beneficial to the participants, as I brought the perspectives of the patient/physician and Lana brought the perspectives of the nurse/primary caregiver/wife to help ensure a robust discussion that would include family members and the stroke survivor.

Most meetings were focused on each participant sharing their story, progress, challenges, and hopes for the future. They also served as a great way to communicate any events happening in our community that would be of interest to our members. The stories shared illustrated a collective never-give-up attitude, and we had many examples of stroke survivors who were still improving years after their stroke had occurred.

New inpatients from the hospital were invited to attend, along with their caregivers and family. This proved especially valuable, as the inpatients were given hope, hearing that that there was life after a stroke as well as witness so many who had gotten better. Equally as important was that the caregivers and families were able to realize they were not alone; there were a lot of stroke survivors who were willing to help simply by sharing their own stories. All in all, this dialogue gave hope to those who needed it most.

Chairing this group was very rewarding to my wife and me. We were able to witness these wonderful conversations and accomplishments every month, and we ensured that everyone in attendance was included in the discussions. We ended up welcoming between twenty and thirty people to the meetings every month, given that unfortunately the incidence of new stroke patients ensured a never-ending influx of new attendees.

Initially, new survivors may be somewhat reluctant to attend survivor meetings, of which many are offered throughout most communities. It is worth attending at least one meeting to meet other survivors, realize you are not alone, and share your concerns and issues with others who have the main benefit of understanding your unique situation and how to better face it. It is also quite motivating to hear the progress others have made. I became a real believer in the value of these meetings after attending just a few.

Initially, I was reluctant to attend, as I really was not interested in hearing other stroke survivor's stories. I believed that I was making good progress and the meetings would not help me. I thought that listening to others might worsen my depression. In hindsight, all these lines of thinking were so wrong. Others' stories motivated me to continue to work hard and to learn about various resources available to stroke survivors in the community. They also kept me up to date on upcoming programs of interest, picnics, walks, and golfing events, all communications that were very welcomed.

As new stroke survivors in the hospital also attended, these meetings provided an excellent opportunity to help address the common concerns new patients have. After all, what better group to do that than one composed of stroke survivors who can show that progress is possible and share how they accomplished their goals! All of this guidance proved so valuable to the new patients and their families while also motivating them to work hard in their own rehab programs and with their therapists. Encouraging new patients not to ever give up was probably the most satisfying part of the meetings for my wife and me, as we believed we were truly helping others to fight on.

We continued to lead the group for five years, at which point I was a bit worn out and felt it was time to give another individual the opportunity to lead and invigorate the group through new ideas and a new perspective. I became a leader emeritus and continued to attend occasional meetings in order to enjoy the camaraderie that exists among stroke survivors. I was always referred to as the founder of the group, which gave me great pride and helped spread awareness of "Dr. K, Stroke Survivor" in the community.

I am happy to report that the group persists and is doing quite well under its current leadership. We still attend from time to time, and I still receive phone calls and emails from new stroke survivors and their families who want little more than to simply talk with another survivor. I help and counsel as much as I am able.

Prior to my departure from VMC, I was asked if I would like to give a brief talk to the staff and patient population from my ward about the work I was doing before I had my stroke. I readily agreed, as it would be a good way to close this particular post-stroke chapter and start a new one through the opportunity to thank everyone for all the work they'd done to help me reach this major milestone. Keeping with my family's celebratory traditions, we made sure a large cake was available for all to eat.

I gave my slide-based presentation while standing at a podium, which really made my therapists happy and proud of how far I had progressed since I was admitted eight weeks earlier. I was asked when I would return for a visit, and I said that I'd be back when I could walk back in, not pushed in a wheelchair. I was leaving in a wheelchair, but I intended to walk through the front doors the next time I visited.

My discharge day arrived, and I was so happy to finally be going home. The aides helped me gather up my belongings and pack them into my car. I transferred from the wheelchair into the front passenger seat, and my wheel-chair was put into the trunk. On the way home, I took in all the sights, realizing that not much had changed—not in terms of scenery anyway. Of course, I cried more of those happy tears as we drove. I felt it was quite miraculous that I had survived the stroke and expended the effort necessary to get better to the point that I could return home as a stroke survivor, not a stroke victim.

CHAPTER TEN

Home At Last

STROKE MYTH

Returning home is easy and requires minimal planning.

Upon returning home, it was hard to fathom that I'd achieved my major goal of surviving the stroke and returning home to my family and familiar surroundings. The walkway that had been installed worked perfectly as a thoroughfare for my wheelchair ride into the house through the backdoor. My daughter had placed a Welcome Home sign over the fireplace hearth in our family room, which was so wonderful to see.

Finally home, I faced new challenges when it came to determining how I would maneuver in my familiar yet strange surroundings. Thankfully, our family room was large enough to accommodate a double bed for my wife and me. I could not believe that I would again be able to sleep with my wife next to me in the same bed. It had been months since we'd been able to do that.

Going anywhere on the first floor required that someone push me in the wheelchair. This was disappointing, but at the same time, there was a big screen TV in the family room that we could watch from our bed, and I had a great view of the backyard where I could see the sky, trees, and our swimming pool. That was the view I awakened to each morning, and it was wonderful. I cherished each new day I woke up. Immediately upon waking, I'd thank God for the gift of another day.

In the evenings, my son or daughter would wheel me into the bathroom so that I could use either the toilet or the shower. I learned how to transfer on and off the toilet as well as into and out of the shower. One of my kids would help me in the shower as needed, although I was able to wash most areas on my own. After showering, I was wheeled back to my bed, where my wife helped me to dress for bed and take my nighttime meds.

As this process developed as our nightly ritual, two problems quickly emerged. The first was that if I had to use the bathroom during the night, I had to wake my wife to help me with a urinal. After a few nights, this was destroying my wife's ability to get a restful night's sleep, so the solution was to place several urinals on a chair next to my side of the bed. That way, I could relieve myself on my own. The second problem was, I sometimes wanted to turn over in bed. While in the hospital, I would just ring for help and someone would appear, help me turn, and place a few pillows behind my back so I would not roll back. As there was no call button at home, I had to wake up my wife to help me, and this added to her lack of sleep. Wearing out a care giver is easy to do, and a solution was needed pronto. It was taking a terrible toll on her strength, and it could not continue.

This problem was solved by my physical therapist, Shelly, who came to my home each week for the next three months. Following discharge from VMC, I was to continue PT and OT at home through an organization called Rehab Without Walls. Insurance allowed for three months of this in-home benefit, after which point, I would have to travel to a rehab out-patient center for longer-term PT and OT.

My new PT was named Shelly, and my OT was named Catherine. I asked Shelly to teach me how to turn over in bed at night without having to disturb my wife. She showed me how to do this, and it worked such that my wife's ability to enjoy a good night's sleep returned. My sleep, however, was now upset by having to pee two to three times per night as well as work to turn in an alternate direction if I wasn't on my back. Since the stroke, I'd been unable to sleep face-down.

During the day, I was wheeled into the kitchen for all meals, and it was wonderful to have homemade meals with my family again. All personal visits were scheduled by my daughter or wife, and they were limited in time so as not to tire me out too much. The effort it required to stay alert, engaged, and able to partake meaningfully in a discussion was terribly unnerving, so these visits were limited by necessity, just as they had been while I was in the hospital. In fact, I occasionally still need to take a nap after a visit from friends!

CAREGIVER CONSIDERATIONS

BY LANA KROCHMAL

Every stroke is unique to the individual who has it. The severity, deficit, and recovery time vary from person to person.

When Lincoln had his stroke, my son, daughter, and I experienced typical feelings of fear, helplessness, anger, disbelief, and finally, acceptance of our situation. Together with the medical and support staff, we developed a plan to help my husband recover his life.

For the first several days following Lincoln's stroke, I was in a state of shock, feeling quite uneasy about how our future would look. It's hard to describe the devastation I felt watching my strong, independent, take-charge husband be swiftly reduced to needing help with everything. He had difficulty speaking, moving, and understanding. I was overwhelmed by all of my new responsibilities, and so sad to see my husband suffering.

With our two adult children at my side, we constructed a plan of action to deal with this new situation. Over the course of the next three months, things did get easier as we adjusted to our new normal and moved forward.

Life has continued to evolve since the stroke, and we have developed ways to enjoy our lives with a bit of a different perspective. Planning has become a necessary exercise when we want to do something outside our usual routine, and a willingness to adjust expectations is of paramount importance.

Support from my wonderful family and our amazing friends has given me the strength and support needed to manage this journey. As they say, "Man plans and God laughs." We never know what the future holds, but I've learned that when the worst happens, don't ask why. Simply accept what is and move forward.

During the past eleven years, we have experienced many ups and downs, but we've always celebrated our progress and our strides forward. Yesterday, today, and tomorrow are a gift. We have, in so many ways, taken our lives back. We hope that in some small way, our story will be of some inspiration and assistance in finding your way after a loved one suffers a stroke.

Over the last eleven years, we've established a list of helpful suggestions to aid the caregiver in navigating their new normal.

1. Adjust your expectations. Stroke recovery is a very slow process.

2. Investigate available resources from social services at the rehab center.

3. Accept help from friends and family when it is offered.

4. Take time for yourself. You will need relief and a diversion from time to time. Caregiving can be exhausting.

5. Emotional support can be helpful. Identify a clergy member or psychologist if necessary to assist you emotionally. It is easy to lose yourself to the act of caregiving.

6. Join a stroke survivors group. You will receive invaluable information from other stroke patients and their families.

7. Accept your new reality. This is your life now. Understand that life does improve and get easier over time.

8. Take your life back. Resume some of the activities you and your family enjoyed before the stroke while realizing that the patient will probably tire easily and need to rest frequently.

CHAPTER ELEVEN

Regaining Freedom at the DMV

STROKE FACT

Regaining your driver's license isn't easy, but it is possible after you reach one year post-stroke.

It's hard to imagine that something truly wonderful can happen at the DMV (Department of Motor Vehicles), but because it was such a significant day in my recovery and serves as proof of what's possible when you put your mind to it, I'll share the story of reclaiming my driving privileges.

When an individual has a stroke, their driver's license is immediately suspended for one year. After a year, you can reapply to get your license back, which initially requires several interviews in order to be cleared to retake the written and driving exams. Losing your license is one of the worst things that happens when it comes to underscoring just how much of your freedom has been lost. You now have to be chauffeured everywhere, for everything, for a year. How depressing and devastating this situation was to me.

As soon as one year had elapsed, I began the application process. The next step was to make an appointment at the DMV for the written and driving tests. My daughter asked if I had practiced driving, and I said yes, but it was limited to backing in and out of my garage a few times. I didn't practice any more than that; I was convinced that I would pass the driving test.

All previous visits to the DMV made me think, "This must be what it's like to visit a leper colony" (no disrespect meant toward those suffering from leprosy). Despite these feelings, however, I marched onward, because getting my driver's license reinstated represented a huge step toward freedom.

My daughter warned me that despite having thoroughly read and highlighted the booklet given to all those wanting to obtain a driver's license, I might fail. My immediate response was, "Failure is not an option." I was going to the DMV to get my license back, and failure be damned; I was going to do it. Once again, my attitude that I would regain as much of my life and independence as possible was alive. It will likely come as no surprise that I passed the written test, and upon successfully passing the driving exam, the evaluator said that I had driven better than most people who had never had a stroke! That produced a huge smile on my face along with some of those aforementioned happy tears. I went back inside to have my picture taken for my license and returned home victorious, victoriously and proudly clutching my license in my right hand. It was a glorious day!

CHAPTER TWELVE

Re-Immersion

STROKE FACT

Rejoining society after a stroke/TBI is critically
important.

I was advised that it was quite important for stroke survivors who had returned home not to lead a reclusive
existence and to avoid becoming hermits. It was critical
to get back out into society. This could be achieved by returning to work (if possible), going shopping, visiting restau-
rants and parties, and doing other things that were part of
one's routine pre-stroke. I had to get used to the inevitable
stares and looks that said, "Poor you" and "I'm so glad it's
not me," and I continued to repeat in my head, "Here but
for the grace of God go I."

Excursions did require some planning, as I had to be
chauffeured wherever I went and helped with transfers in
and out of the car, into and out of the wheelchair, and
pushed around wherever it was that we had gone, as my

ability to walk was quite limited.

That would not change until I not only got my driver's license back but could also transfer into and out of the car on my own and walk a short distance unassisted. It likely goes without saying that this represented a new goal I set out to achieve. Would this process of recognizing new challenges and setting up related goals ever end? No, it would not. That was my lot in life, and I knew I'd better not start feeling sorry for myself. Instead, I needed to channel my energies into continuing to get better and continuing to problem solve.

I attended the annual Golf 4 Life event, which was sponsored by the Pacific Stroke Association and held at the Los Lagos golf course in San Jose for stroke/TBI survivors. I learned about this event through the stroke survivor group meeting and attended for the first time about three years after my stroke and have continued to attend every year since. The first time we went, the event was attended by about eighty survivors and many therapists, nurses, and pro volunteers. The attendees had an opportunity to use the driving range, putting green, or play three holes of golf. Although I was a physician, I had never played golf (other than miniature golf), but I wanted to attend this event to meet other survivors and test my ability to hit a golf ball using only one arm.

What fun I had and how exhilarating was it for me to swing a golf club, feel it hit the ball, and then watch the ball sail through the air for so many yards. Putting and the three-hole course were also great fun. The entire event was closely supervised by the therapists who were always ready to provide assistance. There was a sponsored lunch and a speaker who related his or her stroke history.

In 2014 or 2015, I was asked to be the speaker, and my wife and I were happy to tell our story to all who were assembled. Needless to say, I looked forward to attending this event each September

Some days, this reality was more depressing than others, as it underscored my ongoing dependency on others. Thus, I worked aggressively with my PT to improve my ability to walk and focus on exercises that would strengthen my weak leg. My arm and hand were typically much slower to respond to therapy, however I was slowly able to increase the range of motion in my arm, which made dressing a little easier. My hand was frustratingly slow to improve with therapy, as my goal was to be able to type again on my computer. I was advised that this goal may not be realistic, but I would keep trying, nevertheless.

After three months of therapy at home through Rehab Without Walls, I was ready to continue PT and OT as an outpatient. We decided on Mission Oaks, as they had therapists trained in neuro-IFRAH, which incorporated a special hands-on manipulation in addition to standard therapy. This additional skill was of particular benefit to patients with my specific disability as the result of a stroke.

I attended my first appointment in a wheelchair. I began to have sessions with Kristen (PT) and Carol (OT). They assessed my current state of progress and took baseline measurements, we agreed on goals, and we began weekly therapy. Unfortunately, Medicare only paid for so many sessions per year, so six months in, I was done for the year and would have to wait for another calendar year in order to return. I soon learned that the number of visits per year was the same for a stroke survivor as it was for a patient recovering from a broken limb. I found this to be absolutely ridiculous, but because of my age, I was limited to Medicare insurance.

Once I had become an outpatient, my wife and I volunteered at VMC and Mission Oaks to visit new stroke patients who were in desperate need of help. Lana tended to work with the families and soon-to-be caregivers while I spoke to the patients. I emphasized that not that long ago, I was in the same bed they were in, and I was now walking with a cane and driving again.

This immediately created a predictable bond between survivors, and my credibility was quite high, as the patients knew I understood first-hand what they were going through. Thus, my advice was easily accepted, especially advice that related to having an attitude of not giving up, working hard in therapy, doing one more for good luck, and understanding that emotional lability is part of healing. Over and over, I reminded patients not to fight spontaneous crying, and instead let it out and then get back in the game. I told them that I could not offer them a magic pill or cure, but I could offer them something far more valuable, and that was HOPE!

In order to continue my therapy at home, I hired a caregiver, Marcy, to help me with the exercises assigned by my therapists (who helped train Marcy on how to do them properly). Marcy soon became like a member of the family, helping me when I had to go to a doctor's appointment or to therapy visits, as well as running errands with me to ensure my safety. We became great partners, and she helped me with my mail, organizing my home office, helping me with any projects I undertook, and assisting my wife with some of the chores involved in maintaining the home. Marcy became invaluable to us, and she is still with me after eight years.

CHAPTER THIRTEEN

Bye Bye Wheelchair

STROKE FACT

Eventually getting out of your wheelchair is a major
goal all stroke/TBI survivors strive to achieve.

I began to make good progress walking and doing stairs
with Kristen and then Kristi, another neuro-IFRAH-
trained PT. About six months after beginning therapy at
Mission Oaks, I decided one day that I was doing so well
walking with a cane that the next time I needed to use the
bathroom at home, I would not ask my wife to push me to
the bathroom. I would get up and walk by myself. This was
a very special moment, and I completed my mission successfully. My wife called out, asking what I was doing, and I
responded that I was going to the bathroom. She found me
and was so surprised to see what I had accomplished. For
the first time since the stroke, I was once again able to stand
to urinate and make it back to my chair without falling or
needing assistance. This was huge, as it opened up all kinds

of possibilities: I could stand to shave, brush my teeth, comb my hair, walk into the kitchen for meals, and use toilets when not at home. It may not seem like a big deal to some, but for a man, to be able to stand when urinating is very important. After all, it's a behavior that defines him as a man!

From this point forward, I left my wheelchair behind while at home and walked into and out of Mission Oaks on my own two feet when going for therapy. My therapists were very happy to witness this progress. So, a year after my stroke I was free of the wheelchair and kept it in my car for emergency use or if I was going to be doing something that involved far too much walking.

I was able to walk all around the first floor of my home and climb the stairs to our bedroom, which meant that the family room could return to its original intended use. Continuing to place urinals by my side of the bed ended all disturbance of my wife's sleep.

Returning to my bedroom enabled me to use my own sink and bathroom and to take showers without any assistance from my kids, given that I had a shower bench. The only help I needed was when I exited the shower onto the transport chair and needed to be pushed to my bed. We took this approach in order to avoid having to put my AFO brace and shoes on again.

The next few years focused on my therapy sessions and exploration of anything that might safely speed and aid my recovery.

CHAPTER FOURTEEN

East Meets West

STROKE MYTH

Western medicine's current approach to treating stroke/TBI survivors is all that is available when it comes to hastening one's recovery.

At about the time when I thought I had exhausted every approach Western medicine had to offer, I went to see a movie titled "9000 Needles" about a stroke survivor who went to China for acupuncture after he used up all his health insurance benefits in the US. The film was premiered in Santa Cruz, so my son and daughter took me to see it. The film was made by the patient's brother, whom I had the opportunity to speak with. The story clearly demonstrated that acupuncture helped the patient to move his limbs, walk down stairs, and walk more in general. I decided then that I too would give acupuncture a try.

There are many practitioners of acupuncture in California, and I was able to find one who had been trained in China. I found that this procedure enabled certain muscles in my arm and leg to move for the first time since the stroke while decreasing the stiff muscle tone and pain that I had been experiencing. I continued with these treatments weekly for over a year. In time, I found that their benefit diminished, so I stopped. However, every stroke survivor is different in their response to medication and treatment, and acupuncture was definitely a worthwhile investment. I reasoned "Why not take the best of both Eastern and Western medicine to see if, together, they might benefit me (as long as they are safe)?

Excessive stiff tone in the muscles of my left arm and leg was causing me to have a lot of painful spasms, so I tried various gabapentin medications, which did not help. I also considered a treatment in which I would wear a pump containing baclofen, which would be pumped directly into the intrathecal space around my spinal cord anytime I felt that the spasms were occurring. This was done by implanting a permanent catheter into my spine. I was very reluctant to have this procedure done, because it could be easily dislodged and could also serve as a route for unwanted infection, so I opted to endure the pain rather than take this additional risk.

Another treatment brought to my attention was injections of Botox to relax the muscles. I found a physical medicine and rehab physician who specialized in administering Botox to stroke survivors and underwent injections into the muscles of my arm and leg every three months for two years. Unfortunately, I did not see a dramatic improvement in the spasticity of my muscles. I gave it a try again after a year off, but I had the same outcome. There seemed to be no easy fix in my case.

Also, at the suggestion of my occupational therapist, I decided to spend a week in San Diego at a special clinic with a well-known OT widely considered the father of Neuro-IFRAH. By intensive daily OT and PT therapy, this OT has reportedly helped other stroke survivors make substantial progress in their recovery. In my experience, giving my all each and every day for one week (for eight hours per day, which was painful, difficult, and extremely tiring, I did not achieve the benefit I both hoped for and expected. This was very disappointing, especially given the high cost associated with the program. I concluded that repetitive exercises and ongoing PT/OT with my therapists at Mission Oaks was the best approach when it came to continuing to experience small, incremental improvements.

I looked into hyperbaric oxygen therapy but concluded that the results were mixed and not something I was ready to commit to at the time. I was now several years post-stroke, and this therapy is most effective when given shortly after the stroke occurs. My last great hope was stem cell therapy.

A lot of information related to stem cell therapy for brain damage due to a stroke or TBI can be found on the internet. Clinical trials of stem cells for stroke survivors were being conducted at several well-known medical centers in the US. Upon investigating the enrollment criteria, I discovered that the trials were only open for stroke survivors who'd had clots, not those who had suffered a hemorrhagic stroke, as I did. I could not understand this reasoning, as the impact of damaged brain tissue should be the same regardless of causation. But my reasoning did not matter; after all, I wasn't in charge of the trials.

I was disappointed, given that there were a few reports of patients who had received injection of stem cells directly into their brains at the injury site and had shown dramatic improvement in their ability to use their arms and legs compared to pretreatment. This was most encouraging, so I investigated many places advertising on the internet that they offered stem cell therapy (apart from the approved clinical trials previously mentioned). There were several clinics near our home that offered stem cell therapy at quite a significant cost (to be paid out-of-pocket; insurance was not covering this FDA unapproved treatment). I investigated their reputations and background as well as those of the physicians staffing these clinics. I was encouraged that the clinic I chose utilized the patient's own stem cells, harvested from their abdominal fat via liposuction and then injected into their central nervous system by lumbar puncture. This procedure cost about $20,000, and I thought it would be worth it if my results were similar to those experienced by others.

The scientific data supporting the safety and efficacy of stem cell therapy along with the proposed mechanism of action were substantial and very impressive, as assessed by my own medical training. My post-treatment period was characterized by very uncomfortable sciatic pain in both legs, which lasted for about two days. I had been forewarned that this might be experienced. Fortunately, I had no other side effects, but I also did not enjoy any improvement in the functionality of my arm or leg. About two months later, the stem cell clinic recommended one more treatment using stem cells derived from placental and umbilical cord blood. I decided to give it one more try; despite my commitment to intensive therapy, both PT and OT, I seemed to have leveled off in my overall improvement. The cost of this final treatment was about half of the original fee, and the treatment would be administered intravenously, thus avoiding a repeat of the sciatic pain associated with the first treatment.

I am disappointed to report that this second treatment was also not helpful to me. I felt I had exhausted all reasonable avenues to obtain a breakthrough benefit to my situation. Once again, I recommitted to my usual therapy, working harder and more often at home in between therapy sessions. I would continue to monitor research being done on biomechanics and other areas that might benefit stroke survivors.

I did have an opportunity to try an exoskeleton created by Eksobionics, which was a mechanical, computer-controlled apparatus strapped to the patient to assist with walking. It certainly did work as promised and would be great for new stroke or TBI patients to utilize shortly after their injury in order to show them that it was indeed possible to get up and walk again. I felt this would be tremendously motivating to new patients and would likely speed the process of walking again, providing much earlier independent mobility and discharge from the hospital. To be clear, there was no benefit from this technology for the upper extremity.

I have listed in the appendix all the technologies I tried to help the functionality of my arm and leg along with brief comments as to my experience with each.

CHAPTER FIFTEEN

Where I Stand Today

O nce I began doing the hard work with my therapists and taking some risks that initially seemed daunting, I was determined to get out of my wheelchair as soon as possible. This helped to reestablish my independence and lessoned my reliance on others. I soon discovered that I was even able to do some simple errands on my own, provided I was very careful and engaged in some thoughtful planning ahead of time.

I have continued with my PT and OT therapy as well as aggressively exercising at home, and my walking has continued to improve. I am out in the community frequently, and I drive everywhere! I am pleased to say that my walking has progressed to the point where I am beginning to walk some distances without my cane, which marks the achievement of another major goal. More freedom comes my way! I also believe that my dignity and identity as a physician have, in large part, returned. My next major goal is to strengthen my left ankle so I can do away with my AFO brace and wear my closet full of great shoes that have been patiently waiting for me since 2010.

A few major events have occurred for which I was glad to be around. On July 21, 2012, five years after my stroke, Lana and I had a recommitment marriage to celebrate life after my stroke. It was a wonderful event at which we were surrounded by family and friends.

In 2014, our daughter, Natalie, was married to a local restauranteur. It was a beautiful ceremony up in wine country, north of Sonoma, and I was blessed to be able to walk her down the aisle (a moment that marked the accomplishment of another milestone for me). Then in 2016, we were blessed to have a grandson arrive, and he has really motivated me to continue to work hard on my recovery so I can be a part of his life. I believe this all indicates that I am making the most out of the days I have been blessed to have since the stroke.

All holidays, anniversaries, and birthdays are celebrated and enjoyed, as is watching my favorite sports programs. I spend a large amount of time voraciously reading, knocking off at least one book per week and often reading two or three books simultaneously on my tablet (it is easier for me not to have to hold a physical book and turn pages). There were so many years when I was not reading very much, and I'm now definitely aggressively making up for it. I find that my interests vary considerably between fiction and non-fiction and include books on history, series of books by the same author, biographies, and mysteries.

Writing this book has been another long-term goal of mine. I sure hope it helps other stroke and TBI survivors in dealing with this malady. Another of my everyday goals is to put a smile on my wife's face for saving my life and being such a fantastic caregiver all these years.

I will continue to work on my recovery while knowing that my life won't ever be boring or dull. I aim to enjoy myself as much as I can. As the soul group The Impression's said in their hit song, "Keep on Pushin'." I plan to do just that by continuing to take one step after another and see where it leads me.

Oh, and by the way, I am not disabled. I am:

SORRY

BODY
TEMPORARILY
OUT OF ORDER

TOP 12 DIRECTIVES FOR
STROKE/TBI PATIENTS

- Don't spend a lot of time wondering why you had a stroke.
- Don't waste time feeling sorry for yourself.
- Focus on understanding the impact of the stroke on your mind and body.
- With the input of therapists, define short- and long-term goals as well as a plan to achieve them. Then, execute that plan!
- Assign specific duties and responsibilities to your family members and caregivers.
- Always do one more than you're asked to do when exercising.
- Don't be afraid to take calculated risks. Your therapists are there to give you the tools to have courage and confidence to try.
- Get back out into society—live your life!
- Don't let anyone tell you that you can't do something, If they do, prove them wrong!
- If you fall down, get back up and make sure you never fall again for the same reason.
- In summary, don't let the stroke win. You *can* regain your freedom!
- Think of each new day as a gift.
- Never, never, ever give up!

Appendix

DEVICES TO ASSIST WITH WALKING/HAND FUNCTION
(Discuss these with your therapist, as they can recommend which might be best for your particular situation.)

Bioness
I used the one for the hand, which did stimulate my hand to open, but it requires ongoing support and adjustment by a Bioness technician. The foot drop device unfortunately did not help me.

Saebo
I used and liked the Saebo stretch brace, as it helped with the tone in my hand

The Saebo Glove
This device was also helpful in opening my fingers, allowing me to grip objects.

USEFUL EQUIPMENT
(Each of these items can all be obtained from a general equipment supplier for handicapped individuals.)

- Bedside commode
- Wheelchair
- Transport chair
- Sliding shower bench with a cutout for a good booty

wash

- Traveling shower bench, as most hotels do not have the easiest to use shower benches even in handicap accessible rooms

OTHER RECOMMENDATIONS AND RESOURCES

Books

Healing Into Possibility by Alison Bonds Shapiro

Highs, Lows and Plateaus by Anne Jacobs

After the Stroke: My Journey Back to Life by Mark McEwen

My Stroke of Luck by Kirk Douglas

My Stroke, My Recovery and My Return to the NFL by Tedy Bruschi

My Stroke of Insight by Jill Bolte Taylor

Stroke Recovery Stories by Jeff Kagan

Hope After Stroke for Caregivers and Survivors by T. Tanzman

True Strength: My Journey from Hercules to Mere Mortal and How Nearly Dying Saved My Life by Kevin Sorbo

Stem Cell Therapy
- The Stem Cell Revolution by Berman and Lander
- Stem Cell Therapy by Riordan

Hyperbaric Oxygen Therapy
- The Oxygen Revolution by Harch

Songs that helped cheer me up while at VMC
- "I'm Free" by The Who
- "I'm Still Standing" by Elton John
- "We Gotta Get Out of This Place" by The Animals
- "Keep on Pushing" by The Impressions

Movies or film snippets that made me laugh
- "Dude, Where's my Car" (the Chinese drive-through snippet)
- "Planes, Trains and Automobiles"
- "Uncle Buck"

Brain Games (recommended by speech therapists)
- Lumosity
- BrainHQ

Glossary

ACUPUNCTURE: a key component of Traditional Chinese Medicine that utilizes the insertion of multiple tiny needles in the skin to stimulate nerves to improve circulation, healing and pain. It did help me initially to decrease my pain and allow some muscles to move but the benefit did not persist, despite continued treatments

AFO BRACE: an ankle, foot orthotic brace for providing support for foot drop to prevent dislocation and/or fracture when walking. I have used such a brace since my stroke in 2010.

BACLOFEN: a muscle relaxer and antispasmodic agent. It did not help me.

BIONESS: a company that makes braces or hands and legs that through electrical stimulus can aid functionality. www.bioness.com

BLAIR: a company that makes clothes that are user friendly for stroke or TBI patients. www.blair.com

BOTULINUM TOXIN: works by blocking the signal between

nerves and muscles that makes the muscle contract and tighten. This can provide relief from spasticity symptoms including pain and muscle stiffness. My response has been mixed and I am still undergoing this therapy for my arm and hand, which has the greatest spasticity and pain.

CAT SCAN: uses special X-Rays and a computer to form images and often shows the extent of damage to brain tissue in a stroke. Can also monitor the progression of bleeding in a hemorrhagic stroke.

CEO: Chief Executive Officer, the position I held at the time of my stroke

EKSOBIONICS: the company that has created an exoskeleton to assist a patient with hemiplegia to be able to get up and walk very soon after a stroke or TBI.
www.eksobionics.com

EMT (Emergency Medical Technician): a first responder assigned to an ambulance.

ER (Emergency Room): where all emergency patients are initially brought for evaluation

FOLEY CATHETER: a rubber tube inserted into the bladder to collect urine when it may not be possible for the patient to void on their own

GABAPENTIN: medication to relieve nerve pain.

GURNEY: a wheeled stretcher used for transporting hospital patients

HEMIPLEGIA: paralysis of one side of the body due to a stroke or TBI

HYPERBARIC OXYGEN: a treatment utilizing oxygen under increased pressure to enhance the body's natural healing process by providing an environment which allows the body to absorb much higher amounts of oxygen to all organs of the body including the brain than possible at normal atmospheric pressure. Most helpful if utilized soon after the brain injury (stroke or TBI). I learned of this too late to try.

INTRATHECAL INJECTION: an injection through the spinal cord into the cerebrospinal fluid. Stem cells are administered this way.

MANNITOL: a salty solution given intravenously to increase urine output, thereby decreasing blood volume with the goal of slowing or stopping bleeding in the brain in a hemorrhagic stroke. I was treated with this, and it helped to stop the bleeding in my brain and save my life.

MRI SCAN (Magnetic Resonance Imaging): a special technique in radiology that uses radio waves and a special magnet to form pictures of the anatomical and physiological processes of the body. After a stroke, this imaging can demonstrate the degree of injury to the brain.

NDT (Neurodevelopmental therapy): special hands-on training that PT and OT therapists undergo in order to facilitate and improve movement and mobility in patients with damage to their brain or spinal cord. I made sure all my outpatient therapists had NDT training.

NEUROPLASTICITY: the ability of the brain to adapt to changes in an individual's environment by forming new neural connections over time. It explains how the human brain is able to adapt, master new skills, store memories and information and even recover after a stroke or TBI. Multiple repetitions of an exercise or movement is absolutely a requirement for neuroplasticity to occur.

NEURO-IFRAH: a special training in the treatment and management of patients with hemiplegia from a stroke or TBI emphasizing the restoration of function.

OT (Occupational Therapy): the therapy provided to the arm and hand to help restore functionality and usage

PT (Physical Therapy): the therapy provided to the legs to help restore the ability to walk

RN (Registered Nurse): An RN is different from an LPN (Licensed Practical Nurse) and undergoes far more education and training than an LPN. My wife, Lana, is an RN.

SAEBO: a company that makes many braces and splints for both extremities which can be useful. www.saebo.com

STEM CELLS: undifferentiated cells with the capacity to both differentiate and multiply into the 200 cell types that comprise a human being. There was evidence that stem cell therapy could replace the damaged brain cells. I received one treatment of my own stem cells obtained from my own fat tissue and a second treatment obtained from placental/umbilical cord, neither of which helped in my specific case. It was strictly experimental and fit with my commitment to try safe treatments that might speed my recovery.

TBI: Traumatic Brain Injury such as from blunt traumas in a car crash. Symptoms are similar to those of a stroke, as brain damage often occurs in a TBI.

TPA (Tissue Plasminogen Activator): a treatment administered to those patients who have a stroke from a blood clot. Commonly referred to as a clot buster. Most effective if administered within 3.5 to 5 hours of the stroke.

TYPES OF STROKES: there are basically two types of strokes that can occur to damage brain tissue:
- Hemorrhagic stroke: results from a blood vessel that ruptures, resulting in bleeding into the brain. This is the type of stroke that I experienced.

- Blood clot: a stroke whereby a clot forms somewhere in the body and travels to the brain or forms locally in the brain, resulting in the blockage in the vessel and the death of brain tissue supplied by the blocked vessel.

VMC (Santa Clara Valley Medical Center): has one of the nation's outstanding inpatient rehabilitation centers for treating stroke and TBI patients, where I was for two months after acute treatment at Stanford.

WALK-AIDE: a company that makes brace for hands and legs that through electrical stimulus can aid functionality. www.walk-aide.com

Acknowledgements

I would like to acknowledge my wife, Lana; my son, Noah; my daughter, Natalie; and my son-in-law, Andrew, for their love and support in my recovery.

Thank you to my therapists—Sonia, Shelly, Anne, Kristen, Kristi, Laurie, Hubert, Caroline, Carol, Linda, Amber, and Brian—as well as all my fellow stroke survivors and friends who encouraged me to write this book.

A big thanks to my son, Noah, for his expertise and creativity in designing the cover.

I also wish to thank Elizabeth Lyons, my editor, for providing terrific guidance and professionalism in bringing my story to life.

A special thank you to Dr. Duong, OT/PT.

Also, to Marcy, my in-home caregiver, who has become an integral member of my family as a result of being such an exceptional caregiver!

Love to you all!

About the Author

Lincoln Krochmal, MD (Dr. K.) is a board-certified dermatologist and stroke survivor with more than thirty-eight years' experience in the pharmaceutical and consumer products industries, focusing on the development of new products, both domestically and globally.

His most recent role was as CMO at Neothetics. Inc. (2013-2016). Prior to that he was CEO & President of Excaliard Pharmaceuticals (2008-2010). He successfully led the Excaliard team in generating positive Proof of Concept data for their lead compound as a treatment for reducing skin scarring. This data subsequently resulted in Pfizer acquiring Excaliard in 2011 for a total value of close to $500m.

Prior to that, Dr. Krochmal served as Executive Vice President, Research and Product Development, for Connetics Corporation, a specialty dermatology company headquartered in Palo Alto. Following three and a half years with Connetics, Dr. Krochmal formed his own consultant business, providing strategic guidance and technical assistance to the pharmaceutical and aesthetics industries.

Since suffering his stroke, he has focused on his recovery and, along with his wife, Lana, has volunteered his time providing peer-to-peer counseling to new stroke patients and their families, leading a stroke survivor group at Valley

Medical Center, and serving as a spokesperson for the American Heart Association and the American Stroke Association.

He also continues to be a consultant in Dermatology to the pharmaceutical industry and is presently a member of the Board of Directors for the Children's Skin Disease Foundation. In March 2022, he was awarded a Presidential citation by the American Academy of Dermatology for his career contributions to the specialty and for his volunteerism.

www.POStroke.com

Made in United States
North Haven, CT
12 January 2024

47360764R00071